Carolina Aguilar
Mariana Akemi Nabeshima
Claudio V. Gonçalves

Coffee's effect on viral liver disease

Carolina Aguilar
Mariana Akemi Nabeshima
Claudio V. Gonçalves

Coffee's effect on viral liver disease

The protective effect of coffee on the profile of chronic liver diseases

ScienciaScripts

Imprint

Any brand names and product names mentioned in this book are subject to trademark, brand or patent protection and are trademarks or registered trademarks of their respective holders. The use of brand names, product names, common names, trade names, product descriptions etc. even without a particular marking in this work is in no way to be construed to mean that such names may be regarded as unrestricted in respect of trademark and brand protection legislation and could thus be used by anyone.

Cover image: www.ingimage.com

This book is a translation from the original published under ISBN 978-3-330-75667-0.

Publisher:
Sciencia Scripts
is a trademark of
Dodo Books Indian Ocean Ltd. and OmniScriptum S.R.L publishing group

120 High Road, East Finchley, London, N2 9ED, United Kingdom
Str. Armeneasca 28/1, office 1, Chisinau MD-2012, Republic of Moldova, Europe
Printed at: see last page
ISBN: 978-620-8-27926-4

Summary

CAROLINA SANTIAGO AGUILAR

Frequency of coffee intake in groups of chronic hepatitis B and C patients: The protective effect of coffee on the evolution of chronic hepatopathies

Sao Paulo

Thanks

First of all, I thank God for giving me yet another challenge.

To my family, who have always taught me the importance of studying. I would like to thank my fiancé Fabio Munarin for his patience, understanding and motivation during the years of my master's degree. To my brother-in-law Gustavo Martins for introducing me to clinical research at the Hospital das Clinicas and from then on my journey through the scientific world began.

To my HC family, who have welcomed me since my scientific initiation. Thanks to Helena Scavone Paschoale for her partnership and friendship over the years we worked together, to Mariana Akemi Nabeshima for her willingness to help not only me, but also my colleagues in the little room and whose friendship I will carry with me forever, to Christiane Satie Cobayashi Omosako, Felipe Pereira de Souza, Julia Gloria Lucatelli Pires, Denise Rodrigues Ferreira, Vera Kim and Rodrigo Martins Abreu, Victor Van Vaisberg and Aline Siqueira Ferreira for helping to execute and finalize this work. Claudinha and Dna Fàtima for their help in the secretariat.

To my best friend Claudio Vinicius Gonçalves, who has shared his joys and sorrows with me, as well as helping me with the statistical part of this work. His dedication and patience were essential!

To my advisor, Dr. Suzane Kioko Ono, for showing me the path of education and guiding me through all my work, from my scientific initiation to the completion of my master's degree! Thank you for your dedication, your learning, your motivation, your nudges, your patience and for always believing in me.

Mission given is mission accomplished!

Summary

Aguilar CS. Frequency of coffee intake in groups of chronic hepatopathies infected with hepatitis B and C viruses: The protective effect of coffee on the evolution of chronic hepatopathies [dissertation]. Sao Paulo: University of Sao Paulo, Faculty of Medicine, 2016.

Coffee is one of the most widely consumed drinks in the world and its beneficial effects have been studied for years. As an antioxidant drink, coffee can inhibit liver enzymes, reducing hepatocyte damage and thus having a hepatoprotective effect. This improvement in the liver is directly related to coffee intake. Therefore, this study aims to evaluate the effect of coffee consumption in groups of patients with chronic hepatitis B and chronic hepatitis C, assuming that coffee can slow down the progression of liver damage. Methods: A total of 1169 patients with chronic liver disease were selected from the database of the hepatology outpatient clinic of the Hospital das Clinicas de Sao Paulo, 514 (44%) with hepatitis B virus (HBV) and 655 (56%) with hepatitis C virus (HCV). Variables such as smoking, alcohol consumption, coffee consumption, laboratory tests (ALT, AST, GGT, INR, platelets, total bilirubin, direct bilirubin and indirect bilirubin, albumin and creatinine), APRI and FIB4 to assess fibrosis and the degree of liver damage were taken into account. Results: Through descriptive analysis of the data we observed that 758/1169 (65%) patients consumed coffee. Patients who consumed coffee had lower levels of AST (p=0.004), APRI (p=0.002) and FIB4 (p=0.003). When analyzing by etiology, it was observed that patients with chronic hepatitis C who drink coffee have lower ALT (p=0.021), AST (p=0.005), APRI (p=0.013) and FIB4 (p=0.013) levels and higher albumin levels (p=0.006). The same was not observed for patients with chronic hepatitis B. Conclusions: Coffee intake is associated with a reduction in liver enzymes and seems to be directly linked to a decrease in APRI and FIB4 values in patients with chronic hepatitis C. The same was not observed for patients with chronic hepatitis B. The same is not observed for chronic hepatitis B.

Keywords: coffee, liver cirrhosis, caffeine, hepatitis B, hepatitis C, polyphenols.

1. introduction

Coffee is one of the world's most consumed beverages for its aroma and flavor, and especially for its stimulating effect[1,2] . It has several species, but the most common for commercialization are Arabica and Robusta. A lot has been studied about coffee in order to assess the beneficial effects that this ancient drink can have on our bodies. Both the beans and the drink have various elements in their composition. Antioxidants, sugars, lipids and amino acids are some of the components present, which can vary in concentration according to the processing of the beans, the species and the type of preparation .[3]

Caffeine and antioxidants are the main elements present in the beans. Caffeine undergoes the action of liver enzymes and is transformed into theobromine and theophylline, which are paraxanthines and will be involved in the liver detoxification process. As well as bioactive compounds which are antioxidants and reduce intracellular oxidative stress[4,5] . Recent studies show that frequent coffee consumption is associated with a decrease in liver enzymes[6-8] , a decrease in cellular oxidation through antioxidant agents[9,10] , as well as a decrease in the risk of hepatocellular carcinoma .[9, 11, 12]

For years, coffee has been the subject of research and its beneficial effects have been thoroughly analyzed in order to clearly understand each mechanism of action. In Brazil, few studies have analyzed the properties of this beverage on liver function. Therefore, this study aims to analyze the progression of liver disease in the presence or absence of coffee, as well as the profile of the coagulation system of patients treated at the Hepatology Outpatient Clinic of the Hospital das Clinicas of FMUSP.

1.2 Coffee composition

Coffee, from the *Rubiaceae* family*, is* a fruit of the *Coffea* genus *and* has several species, the best known being Arabica and Robusta (Canephora). It is one of the world's most widely consumed beverages, with the *Arabica* species being the most characteristic in Europe, America and South India. The species have different biochemical compositions, with Arabica having more trigonelline and Robusta more caffeine[1 3]. In general, they have a stimulating character, as they contain caffeine, as well as tannins and essential oils which give the drink its distinctive aroma.

The raw coffee bean is made up of skin (exocarp), pulp (endocarp), mucilage (mesocarp), parchment (spermoderm) and seed (endosperm). When coffee is processed, the pulp is obtained, which represents around 29% of the dry weight of the whole fruit; 76% water, 10% protein, 2% fiber, 8% ash and 4% nitrogen-free extract, represented by tannins, pectic substances, reducing and non-reducing sugars (^{3}), caffeine, chlorogenic acid and caffeic acid, cellulose, hemicellulose, lignin, amino acids, minerals such as potassium, calcium, iron, sodium, magnesium and others[5] -.

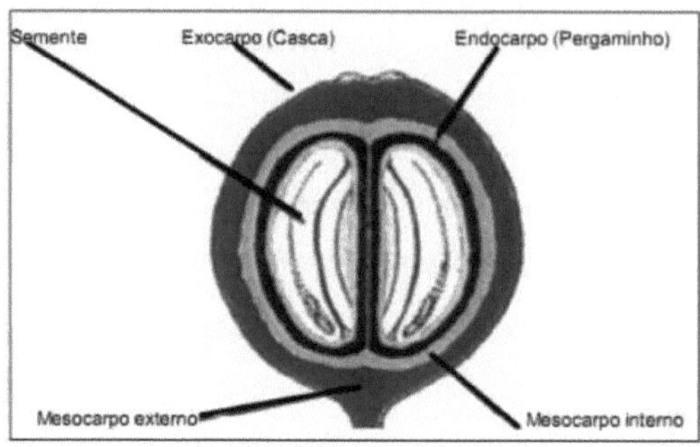

Figure 1 - Cross-sectional composition of raw coffee beans[14]

Coffee beans contain 0.9 to 2.4% caffeine ,[15][16] and the amount can vary according to the species[2] . Caffeine is a xanthine alkaloid and is rapidly absorbed in the intestine, being almost 100% bioavailable and distributed to the tissues. After ingestion, the pyosmotic concentration of caffeine can be observed 30 to 60 minutes after oral administration. Caffeine can be found as the active ingredient in plants such as mate tea, coffee, cocoa, guarana, chocolate, soft drinks and energy drinks and is consumed in the form of infusions .[17]

Coffee beans contain approximately sixty bioactive components, which we call chlorogenic acids (CGAs) and derived compounds([1] 8) where caffeoylquinic, dicaffeoylquinic, feruloylquinic, p-coumaroylquinic acids and mixed esters of caffeic, ferulic and quinic acids are found in the main groups of chlorogenic acid with at least three isomers in each group. They are present in greater quantities in the grains and have antioxidant characteristics ([1] 5, ,[1920]). The chemical composition of raw Arabica beans is 1.2g100g^{-1} of caffeine, 1.0g100g^{-1} of trigonelline, 6.5g100g^{-1} of chlorogenic acids and 16g100g^{-1} of lipids; while robusta beans have 2.2g100g^{-1} , 0.7g100g^{-1} , 10100g^{-1} g and 10g100g^{-1} respectively .[16]

Coffee beans, raw or roasted, have fatty elements present in the endosperm and are made up of triacylglycerols (81.1%), fatty acids (1.6%) and a fraction of diterpenes (17.3%) called cafestol and kahweol[21] . These compounds have been described in the literature as having an anti-carcinogenic biological effect[22,23] and having a hepatoprotective effect against the genotoxic effect of aflotoxin B1 on the hepatocytes of animals and humans[24] . In preparations where the coffee is filtered through a paper filter, there is a reduction in the

6

concentration of these lipids, since most of them are retained on the paper and a small part remains in the drink, which can discreetly raise the levels of total cholesterol and LDL-cholesterol without a significant risk. This risk increases in preparations where the coffee is not filtered, such as espresso, but more studies are needed for clearer proof .[25]

Caffeine is the most stable component, as it doesn't undergo significant degradation[26] , and remains in practically the same quantities before and after roasting[27]. The grind of the bean also affects the quality of the drink, as the higher the degree of grind, the longer it takes for the water to pass through the powder and the greater the extraction of the compounds.

Decaffeinated coffee is produced by chemical extraction [2] , but the caffeine is not completely removed, a residual value of 0.1% is found in the beans, which is accepted by Brazilian legislation[15] which corresponds to approximately 3mg per cup [28], but as caffeine is thermostable and difficult to remove, with extraction, many bioactive compounds end up being lost in this process .[29]

1.3 Roasting and grinding coffee beans

The quality of coffee is defined by the physical characteristics of the beans and the sensory characteristics of the drink. High-temperature roasting can increasingly degrade the bioactive compounds, also known as polyphenols, present in the beans and compromise their antioxidant effect, as the high temperature causes the appearance of free radicals [30,31] . The intensity of the temperature and the roasting time cause the chlorogenic acids present in coffee beans to be degraded[32] , thus forming other compounds, such as nicotinic acid, and up to 90% of the CFAs can be lost[16,33] . This is why it is important to choose the right temperature and time to maintain their sensory qualities[34].

A study of *Coffea Arabica* coffee beans tested the sensory quality of coffee roasted at three different times T1, T2 and T3 (7, 9 and 11 minutes respectively) at the same temperature (95-98°C). After roasting, the coffee was filtered for analysis of taste, aroma and acidity. The author describes that the best sensory quality of the coffee was at time T2 and that these characteristics may be closely linked to chlorogenic acids and the degradation of trigonelline .[35]

The grind of the beans also affects the amount of antioxidants extracted during the preparation of the drink. The finer the grind, the fewer free radicals are present, because the freeze-drying process of finely ground coffee means that these radicals are largely extracted in this process[30].

1.4 Types of preparation

There are different ways of preparing coffee, and in each case the amount of polyphenols can be different. According to the Minas Gerais State Coffee Industry Union, the preparation is classified as follows: weak (70g of powder), medium (70g to 90g of powder) and strong (100g of powder) for 100ml of water[36] . When preparing coffee, some basic rules are used to maintain the sensory characteristics. The substrates must be extracted with hot water at a temperature of 90-100°C without boiling. This process is called infusion and can be done by filtering, percolation, pressing or pressure[37] . The type of coffee preparation influences the quantity of compounds. In percolation, the levels of products from the degradation of trigonelline are higher ([19]), while in filtering the coffee, the porosity of the paper, the time and temperature of extraction and the degradation of the compounds during roasting can interfere with these quantities .[25]

According to the ABIC website, the definitions of the types of preparation are listed below:

When filtering, the powder is added to a paper or cloth filter and hot, non-boiling water is poured on top. This method is used in Brazilian culture in home-made strainers and electric coffee makers.

In percolation, the powder and water are placed in a *moka* pot and placed directly on the stove. The boiling water presses the liquid coffee into the container above. This is the most widely used way of drinking coffee in Europe.

When pressing, the powder is placed in a glass container with non-boiling water and then a filter is inserted and pressed by a plunger which separates the powder from the finished coffee. This method is also known as the French press and is widely used by North Americans.

In the espresso method, the coffee is freshly ground and placed in a filter that is pressurized with water at 90°C and 9 kg of pressure for an average of 30 seconds, producing a creamy, aromatic drink. Created by the French, espresso is considered the most appropriate method for appreciating all the nuances of this drink ([3] 7).

1.6 Function, metabolism and action of antioxidants

Reactive oxygen species (ROS) and reactive nitrogen species (RNS) are products of cellular metabolism and have beneficial effects in low and moderate concentrations that defend organisms against infectious agents. An excess of these products is called free radicals, which cause biological damage called oxidative stress and nitrogen stress. Certain habits determine the appearance of ROS, such as diet, alcohol consumption, physical activity, obesity and other stressors(38, .[39])

Free radicals can be defined as molecules or molecular fragments that contain one or more electrons in the atomic or molecular orbit that trigger metabolic processes by binding with an oxygen molecule forming a superoxide anion radical (O_2^-) and nitric oxide (NO) that interact with other molecules generating other reactive oxygen and/or nitrogen species. Exposure to these free radicals causes the body to develop defense mechanisms to prevent and repair possible damage to cells called antioxidants, which can be enzymatic (superoxide dismutase, glutathione peroxidase and catalase) and non-enzymatic (ascorbic acid, beta-tocopherol, glutathione, carotenoids, flavonoids and others). ROS are also responsible for triggering the carcinogenic process by inducing the DNA of normal cells to transform into tumor cells. Experimental tests indicate that coffee can interfere with different stages of cancer[39] . Xanthine oxidase is an example of a catalytic enzyme that forms ROS and is present in the metabolism of purines, oxidizing xanthines to uric acid .[40]

The protective biotransformation of aromatic hydrocarbons, which takes place mainly in the liver and stomach, is carried out by a series of enzymes called cytochrome P450 monoxygenase/oxy-reductase, as they absorb UV rays at 450nm. These enzymes reduce aromatic hydrocarbons to monoxides, as they have the function of carrying out oxidations and detoxifications and have remaining characteristics using the same basic mechanism, although each enzyme adapts to a structural chemical group. These detoxifications transform active pharmacological compounds into inactive ones to be excreted in the urine, but they also participate in metabolic activation, causing poorly reactive compounds to be transformed into toxic compounds .[41, 42]

1.6.1 Cytochrome P450 (CYP1A2)

In addition to catalyzing reactions, the cytochrome P450 (CYP) enzyme participates in the metabolism of exogenous substrates such as drugs, pro-carcinogens, organic solvents, among others, and endogenous substrates such as cholesterol, bile acids and fatty acids. It also functions as an important defense mechanism against unknown molecules and is present in different tissues, but is most active in the liver(41, 42). CYP1A2 represents 13% of all these enzymes in the liver and can inhibit or induce reactions. In inhibition, the enzyme's activity decreases and there is an accumulation of xenobiotics or drug concentration, intensifying its action(43). CYP induction leads to less exposure to xenobiotics, accelerating the elimination of metabolites or faster elimination of drugs, thus reducing the concentration of the drug in vivo.

Caffeine, for example, inhibits the expression of hepatocyte connective tissue growth factor by increasing the concentration of cyclic adenosine monophosphate (cAMP) which leads to increased degradation of tumor growth factor (TGF-beta) which directly interferes with the enzymes Smad2 and Smad3 .[44, 45]

Caffeine and the acids present in coffee, when ingested, act as antioxidants and are therefore used as biomarkers to assess the reduced risk of a disease, such as type 2 diabetes mellitus. Each of these biomarkers has a different half-life, which can vary between 30 - 480 minutes, but their presence can be seen in both the bloodstream and urine even 8 hours after ingesting the infusion. The peak concentration of caffeine and caffeic acid after ingestion is approximately 60 minutes, and they are therefore considered to be rapidly absorbed, but frequent moderate ingestion of the drink keeps these levels constant and reinforces the idea that there is detoxification of cells and induction of the activity of phase II expression enzymes .[4, 19]

Although some studies don't specify the amount in ml of coffee ingested, Higdon (2006) says that one cup of coffee contains 85-100mg of caffeine and according to Abraham (1997) the ideal consumption of coffee, considered moderate, is 2-3 cups a day([1]). Excessive use (5-6 cups a day) can lead to toxicity, mainly due to the excess of theobromine, which is the main active metabolite in caffeine([46]). According to the European Food Information Council (EUFIC), the average caffeine content of 150 ml (one cup) of ground roasted coffee is around 85 mg, instant coffee 60 mg, decaffeinated coffee 3 mg, leaf tea or sachets 30 mg, instant tea 20 mg and cocoa or hot chocolate 4 mg. A glass (200 ml) of caffeinated soft drink contains between 20 and 60 mg of caffeine ([8] ,).[47]

A study by Yen *et al* (2005) showed that the greater the amount of residues present in roasted coffee, the greater its antioxidant action. In this study, the coffee samples were diluted in ethanol and boiling water. The extraction of roasted coffee residues with the solvents showed that the yield with water was 6.58% and with ethanol 1.38% and, with this, it was possible to observe that coffee can be used as a potent natural antioxidant[32] .

1.7 Health effects of coffee

Despite the antioxidant effect, an exacerbated intake of polyphenols can cause some adverse effects, such as having carcinogenic/genotoxic effects caused by high doses or concentrations added to the diet, interfering with the biosynthesis of thyroid hormones in the inhibition of thyroid peroxidase by some flavonoids, antinutritional effect in the inhibition of non-heme iron absorption resulting in increased iron depletion and interaction with certain pharmacological agents where inhibition of CYP3A4 occurs .[48]

According to Abraham (1997) caffeine can reduce the risk of various types of cancer, and has a stimulating effect on the heart, nervous system and kidneys, as well as stimulating intestinal peristalsis and being used against dehydration[49] in the case of diarrhea, but it is contraindicated in children as it exacerbates the activity of the nervous system ([1]). The drink can reduce cholesterol, bile acids and serve as an antioxidant[50] as well as being beneficial in reducing the risk of various diseases such as cardiovascular diseases and cancers .[51]

Cano-Marquina (2013) in his meta-analysis identified the impact of coffee on health. Her survey from 1990 to 2012 showed that coffee has a beneficial effect not only on the liver, but also on reducing the risk of type 2 diabetes, cardiovascular disease, Parkinson's disease and other neurological disorders, as well as reducing the risk of cancer depending on the tissue affected. Although much has been said about coffee and the risk of osteoporosis, more studies are needed to prove this interaction .[8]

1.7.1 Coffee and cardiovascular disease

On the risk of cardiovascular disease and coffee consumption, a meta-analysis showed that until the 1960s, studies pointed to an increase in arrhythmia associated with coffee consumption. By the 2000s, this association had changed, showing that the risk is directly proportional to excessive coffee consumption, just like smoking. Moderate coffee consumption in patients at risk of cardiovascular disease has shown that the risk is low in these cases .[52]

The relationship between coffee intake and the risk of hypertension by Uiterwaal (2007) evaluated coffee consumption and hypertension. This study showed that only those who did not drink coffee, women and those who drank an excessive amount of coffee (>6 cups/day) were at low risk. The analysis was carried out using a questionnaire which included how many cups of coffee each individual drank a day, the type of coffee (regular, decaffeinated, other) and whether they added other components to the coffee such as milk, sugar or others. The statistical analysis compared individuals with and without hypertension and came to the conclusion that the highest number of individuals without hypertension was observed in those who consumed more than 6 cups of coffee a day in men, and 3-6 cups a day in women. The lowest number of individuals with hypertension was found in women who consumed 3-6 cups of coffee a day .[53]

1.7.2 Coffee and liver disease

It is well known that alcohol consumption alters the GGT enzyme in the liver, but a study carried out in Finland[7] showed that the consumption of 5 cups of coffee or more a day, in individuals who consume 280g of ethanol a week, decreases the levels of the enzyme in 50% of men and women compared to those who don't drink coffee. When drinking 3-4 cups a day, the decrease in levels is smaller, but still significant. This association occurs because when alcohol is consumed at high levels, glutathione is not synthesized and consequently the increase in oxidative stress leads to hepatotoxicity.

Other authors have shown that the progression of necroinflammation together with alcohol and tobacco abuse is not related when caffeine is ingested; necroinflammation can decrease independently of these external factors. This relationship is only positive when alcohol abuse is compared with cigarette abuse, in which case the progression of liver fibrosis is greater[5 4,55] . However, the consumption of alcoholic beverages can hinder the action of bioactive compounds and thus the hepatic protective effect is null[5 6].

In liver cirrhosis, whether alcoholic or non-alcoholic, a protective effect can be observed, as the levels of gamma glutamyltransferase, alanine aminotransferase (ALT) and asparate aminotransferase (AST) were decreased with the intake of 1 cup of coffee per day resulting in a significant reduction in the risk of hepato-cell carcinoma compared to non-drinkers[6, 57] . Another study shows that coffee can also protect the liver against the effects of hepatitis C, but some patients may have their coffee consumption reduced due to impaired caffeine metabolism or medical advice[58] . In patients with untreated hepatitis C, caffeine intake may reduce hepatic necroinflammation and slow the progression of fibrosis .[54]

Liver fibrosis was studied in human and rat liver cells and it was shown that coffee intake can reduce this progression. Human cells were cultured *in vitro* with 1mmol, 5mmol and 10mml of caffeine at 24h and 48h; and tested on 21 cirrhotic rats who were divided into 3 groups and monitored for 8 weeks. This study, carried out by Shim *et al* (2013), showed a direct effect on liver cells. There was a decrease in the progression of fibrosis over a longer period of exposure of human liver cells to caffeine, however the dose of caffeine for the antifibrotic effect has not been well defined .[59]

The effect of the components present in coffee can be observed in the study by Arauz (2013) who evaluated the antifibrotic properties of coffee with and without caffeine in liver cells of rats induced to cirrhosis and also observed the enzyme levels ALT, GGT and Alkaline Phosphatase which decreased significantly in the presence of coffee with or without caffeine. Liver tissue necrosis was attenuated in the presence of coffee regardless of the presence of caffeine and the author concluded that caffeine was not related to the beneficial effect .[60]

Another study in rats showed that paraxanthine (1,7-dimethylxanthine), which comes from caffeine, is a potent inhibitor of the tumor factor TGF-β and that its effect is also due to the presence of caffeine (1,3,7-trimethylxanthine) on the progression of chronic liver fibrosis[45] . This is shown by Modi *et al* (2010) in HCV patients who consumed more than 308mg of caffeine daily and had a reduction in fibrogenic activity compared to non-coffee drinkers .[61]

In patients with liver cirrhosis and viral hepatitis, the rate of caffeine release is lower and the degree of liver dysfunction can therefore be assessed, as caffeine is suggested for testing liver dysfunction due to its relative lack of toxicity, rapid absorption and complete biotransformation by cytochrome P450-dependent liver monooxygenase. One study evaluated 26 patients with liver cirrhosis, 37 with chronic hepatitis and 20 healthy volunteers who received oral doses of 300mg of caffeine dissolved in water. Blood tests were taken after 4, 8 and 12 hours. It was observed that caffeine excretion was lower, around 60%, in cirrhotic patients compared to healthy volunteers[62] . In viral liver cancer, there is less alcohol intake and more coffee intake, so ALT levels are lower and disease progression improves ([63-66]).

In viral hepatitis, studies have suggested that coffee can inhibit viral replication in both *in vitro* and *in vivo* models[56] . There are few studies on Hepatitis B, most involve the C virus, but it is known that coffee compounds (especially caffeic acid) can inhibit the spread of the virus even in the presence of antivirals such as Peginterferon or Ribavirin[67] , because even if patients taking antivirals do not respond to treatment, there is still an inverse association with coffee intake and the progression of liver disease .[68]

In hepatitis B, the effect of coffee has not yet been clearly established. Alcohol intake is evident in this population and directly proportional to coffee intake[69] , but alcohol hinders the action of coffee and worsens fibrosis and cirrhosis.

Wang (2009) showed in a culture of HepG2 liver cells that hepatitis B virus (HBV) replication can be inhibited by the chlorogenic acids present in coffee with or without caffeine. The cells were treated with chlorogenic acids (CGAs) present in coffee, specifically quinic and caffeic acid. DNA was extracted and then quantified using the PCR method. Treatment with antivirals was used as a positive test. The results showed that AGCs had an inhibitory effect on HBV viral replication and DNA levels in the cytoplasm also decreased(7).[0]

1.7.3 Coffee and type 2 diabetes

Studies have shown that coffee intake reduces the risk of type II diabetes. In diabetic rats with metabolic syndrome that received daily doses of coffee for 30 days, there was a decrease in glucose levels, triglycerides, total cholesterol and fractions, creatine, uric acid and hepatic enzyme activity[71] . In a randomized clinical study of 33 patients, 16 of whom were eutrophic and 17 obese/overweight, who received 200ml of instant coffee (3 to 6mg/kg) or water after a meal, it was found that insulin and glucose levels increased within 30 minutes of the meal, after which time the levels returned to normal values. In overweight/obese patients these levels were significantly higher compared to eutrophic patients, but the insulin peak could be observed in 30 minutes in patients who received water or 3mg of coffee and 60 minutes in those who received 6mg, which resulted in a postponement of the drop in glucose concentration subsequently[72] . Patients with type II diabetes and liver fibrosis who have severe non-alcoholic steatohepatitis have an inverse relationship with coffee consumption, as lower insulin resistance has a lower risk of advancing fibrosis, and coffee consumption with a high HOMA-IR index shows no protective effect on advanced fibrosis [73]

Coffee intake and type II diabetes is higher in women, non-smokers and individuals with a normal BMI ($<25kg/m^2$). The incidence of type II diabetes decreases by 12% with every 2 cups a day, 11% with every 2 cups of decaffeinated coffee and 14% with every 200mg of caffeine ingested a day[7 4]. A study of healthy young adult men showed that both decaffeinated and caffeinated coffee attenuate hepatic insulin resistance and even with a higher glucose supplementation load there is no increase in intrahepatic lipids .[8]

1.7.4 Coffee and cancer

A meta-analysis carried out in 2014 looked at the association between coffee consumption and certain types of cancer, such as breast, prostate, colon, liver and rectum. It found that in the case of breast cancer, many studies are still needed, as there was an inverse relationship between coffee intake and a lower risk of cancer in the post-menopause and there was no relationship with the consumption of a cup of coffee. In hepatocellular carcinoma, the relationship with coffee is inversely significant for high coffee consumption, but the survey shows that the hepatocellular carcinoma studies are carried out in Asia where coffee consumption is not common .[39]

Some authors have published on the effects of coffee on health. According to Bravi *et al* (2007) some compounds in coffee can act by blocking agents via modulation of enzymatic multiplication involved in carcinogenic detoxification. They can also modify xenotic metabolism via induction of glutathione-S-transferase and inhibition of *N-acetyltransferase*. In this study, cirrhotic patients and hepatitis B and C virus carriers in southern Europe and Japan were divided into 3 different groups according to the amount of coffee they drank. The results showed that in patients who drank more than 3 cups a day, the risk of hepatocellular carcinoma decreased compared to those who never drank coffee. A meta-analysis carried out by the same author on liver cancer showed that coffee compounds act on enzymes that indicate severe liver disease (ALT), and coffee is therefore inversely associated with the disease. In cases of hepatocellular carcinoma, several studies have shown the beneficial effect of coffee consumption and concluded that there is a 40% lower risk compared to non-coffee drinkers. This effect can be observed because it is known that coffee affects liver enzymes and the development of cirrhosis .[75]

Studies also show the influence of coffee in reducing the progression of liver diseases such as cirrhosis, hepatitis C and hepatocellular carcinoma. According to Inoue (2005), men and women who drink coffee every day have a lower risk of HCC than those who don't drink coffee. The authors speculate that this is due to the action of coffee inhibiting the activity of gamma glutamyltransferase (GGT) and thus the liver would be protected against cell damage due to alcohol .[57]

Considering that coffee is a widely consumed beverage in our country, it has been speculated that the substances in its content may affect liver metabolism and thus modify the natural history of chronic liver disease. The aim of this study is therefore to review current knowledge on the effect of coffee on liver disease and to evaluate coffee consumption in groups of chronic liver disease patients with or without cirrhosis, with the hypothesis that coffee consumption may have a protective effect by inhibiting enzymatic activity in the liver.

2. Objectives

2.1 General Objective

To evaluate the intake of coffee in groups of chronic hepatitis B and C patients, with the hypothesis that its consumption may have a hepatoprotective effect.

2.2 Specific Objectives

To analyze the levels of hepatocellular enzymes, platelets, FIB4 index and APRI in patients who drink coffee or not according to the etiology of their liver disease (HBV or HCV).

3. Methods

This is a prospective, observational, cross-sectional, epidemiological study aimed at analyzing coffee intake in chronic liver disease patients with hepatitis C virus who attended the Clinical Hepatology Outpatient Clinic of the Hospital das Clinicas of the USP School of Medicine and who answered a questionnaire with questions related to habits such as smoking, alcohol consumption, medication use and coffee intake. A bibliographic review was carried out in PubMed and Embase of the last 10 years on the effects of coffee on liver health and the findings were compared with the analyses in this study.

3.1 Patients

Patients were consecutively selected from the database of the hepatology outpatient clinic at Hospital das Clinicas FMUSP using the following inclusion criteria: over 18 years of age, both sexes, patients with hepatitis B virus (AgHBs +) or hepatitis C virus (Anti-HCV + and PCR +), cirrhotic and non-cirrhotic and who signed the Informed Consent Form. The exclusion criteria were: patients with other liver diseases, HIV-positive, co-infected with hepatitis B and C, patients with missing questionnaire data or incomplete laboratory tests.

3.2 Laboratory Analysis

To analyze liver function and damage, Alanine Aminotransferase (ALT), Asparate Aminotransferase (AST), Gamma Glutamyltransferase (GGT), Alkaline Phosphatase (AF), Thrombin Time and INR (TP-INR), Platelets (PLAQ), Total Bilirubin (BT), Direct Bilirubin (BD), Indirect Bilirubin (IB), Albumin (ALB) and Creatinine (CRE) were collected through the Hospital Information and Management System - SIGH of the Hospital das Clinicas de Sao Paulo using only the first blood collection carried out by the hospital.

For the diagnosis of liver cirrhosis, the AST- to-platelet ratio index (APRI) and Fibrosis-4 (FIB-4)[76-79] were used as a non-invasive assessment tool.

3.3 Questionnaires

Coffee intake was assessed by means of a questionnaire in which patients answered about their habit (not drinking or drinking coffee) and the volume of coffee drunk per day (0, 50, 100, 150, 180 or more than 180mL) and this volume was then stratified into not drinking coffee, drinking <100ml and ≥100ml . Other information about other foods and drinks containing caffeine (energy drinks, tea, soft drinks, chocolate, guarana extract and coffee with milk) and decaffeinated coffee was not taken into account, as well as the brands and types (brewed, espresso, short) of coffee consumed.

Other habits are also described in the questionnaire, such as drinking and smoking. Patients who answered yes or no to the questions related to the consumption of alcoholic beverages and tobacco were considered for this study; those who answered "former drinker" or "former smoker" were not considered in the analysis. The amount of alcohol consumed or the number of cigarettes per day were not analyzed. The same was done for the medications; it was not established what type of antiviral medication was administered or the length of treatment, only whether or not there was treatment with antivirals.

The questionnaires and the database come from the research project "Frequency of the UGT1A1*28 allele in patients with chronic liver disease and in healthy controls" CAPPesq 056/06, session 23.02.06. All the questionnaires were applied after signing the Informed Consent Form.

3.4 Statistical Analysis

The data was presented as median and interquartile range (Q1 - Q3) for quantitative variables and as absolute frequency and percentage for qualitative variables. To check for associations between qualitative variables, the chi-square test with Yates correction was used for 2 x 2 tables and the chi-square test when one of the variables had more than two categories. To compare means between two independent groups, the Mann-Whitney U-test was used; to compare means between three or more independent groups, the Kruskal-Wallis test followed by Tamhane was used as a *post-hoc* test. All tests were two-tailed and the significance level adopted was 5%. The analyses were carried out using the Statistical Package for Social Sciences (SPSS) software version 13.0 for Windows (Chicago, IL, United States).

4. Results

Table 1 shows the demographic characteristics of the patients selected for the study. The study included 1,169 patients with a mean age of 58±14 years, of whom 588 were male (50%) and 581 female (50%). The percentage of smokers and alcohol intake were higher in males ($p < 0.001$). In terms of etiology, the majority of patients were diagnosed with the hepatitis C virus (56%). The analysis between genders showed that women had a higher percentage of this virus (348/581, 60%) while men had a higher percentage of the hepatitis B virus (281/ 588, 48%), but the differences were not significant ($p = 0.10$).

Less than half of all patients treat or have treated their illnesses with antivirals (45%), and 65% of them report drinking coffee.

Table 1 - Patients' general characteristics

	Total n 1169	(%) (100%)	Men n 588	(%) (50%)	Women N 581	(%) (50%)	p
Age (years + SD)	58 ± 14		58 ± 14		60 ± 14		0,004
Smokers	212	(18%)	123/588	(21%)	89/581	(15%)	< 0,001
Alcohol intake	182	(16%)	101/588	(17%)	81/581	(14%)	< 0,001
Etiology							
HBV	514	(44%)	281/588	(48%)	233/581	(40%)	0,10
HCV	655	(56%)	307/588	(52%)	348/581	(60%)	
Use of antivirals	528	(45%)	271/588	(46%)	257/581	(44%)	0,563
Coffee intake	758	(65%)	394/588	(67%)	364/581	(63%)	0,134

When we analyzed the characteristics of the 1,169 patients according to etiology (Table 2), we could see that alcohol intake was higher in Hepatitis B patients and was statistically significant (n= 96, 19%, *p= 0.029*). Coffee intake was also higher in this group, but was not statistically significant. The number of patients taking antivirals was higher in the C virus group (Table 2).

Table 2 - General characteristics of patients according to etiology

	Total		Hepatitis B		Hepatitis C		
	N	(%)	n	(%)	n	(%)	
	1169	(100%)	514	(44%)	655	(56%)	p
Age (years + SD)	50 ± 14		55 ± 14		61	± 13	< 0,001
Smokers	212	(18%)	84	(16%)	128	(20%)	0,217
Alcohol intake	182	(16%)	96	(19%)	86	(13%)	0,029
Use of antivirals	528	(45%)	201	(39%)	327	(50%)	< 0,001
Coffee intake	758	(65%)	343	(67%)	415	(63%)	0,256

Table 3 shows the laboratory profile of all the patients separated by etiology. Statistical significance was observed in the liver enzymes ALT, AST and GGT for the B virus, which had lower median values than the C virus. AST and GGT were also lower in the B virus when compared to all patients (p < 0.001 for all comparisons).

Platelets showed a better level in the B virus patients compared to the HCV group (mean 179.9 ± 83.7 vs 154.3 ± 85 x10^3/mm^3 , *p= 0.001*). This was also reflected in the evaluation of the APRI and FIB4 indices, which showed statistically significant lower levels in the hepatitis B group compared to the C virus group (p < 0.001 for both comparisons).

Table 3 - laboratory aspects according to etiology

	Total n= 1169 (100%)					Hepatitis B n = 514(44%)					Hepatitis C n= 6î 55 (56%)					P
	average	DP	25%	Median	75%	average	DP	25%	Median	75%	average	DP	25%	Median	75%	
ALT (UI/L)	72,5	+ 191,1	26,0	42,0	75,0	74,5	+ 273,0	20,0	31,0	57,8	70,9	+ 82,6	33,0	53,0	83,0	<0,001
AST (UI/L)	67,7	+ 155,5	26,0	40,0	68,0	66,9	+ 203,6	22,0	30,0	50,0	68,3	+ 103,2	32,0	49,0	76,0	<0,001
FA (UI/L)	98,2	+ 54,2	65,5	83,0	113,0	96,5	+ 52,4	65,0	81,0	107,8	99,6	+ 55,6	67,0	84,0	114,0	0,108
GGT (UI/L)	90,1	+ 110,9	26,0	52,0	103,0	76,8	+ 105,5	21,0	40,0	80,0	100.5	+ 113,8	34,0	60,0	124,5	<0,001
PLAQ (mil/mm)^3	170,3	+ 87,7	97,0	170,0	228,0	179,9	+ 83,7	124,3	183,0	232,0	162,8	+ 90,1	190,0	153,0	221,5	<0,001
TP-INR	1,1	+ 0,3	1,o	1,1	1,2	1,1	+ 0,2	1,o	1,1	1,2	1,1	+ 0,2	1,0	1,1	1,2	0,496
ALB (g/dL)	4,2	+ 0,6	3,9	4,3	4,6	4,2	+ 0,6	4,0	4,4	4,6	4,2	+ 0,6	3,9	4,3	4,5	0,002
BT (mg/dL)	1,3	+ 2,5	0,6	0,8	1,2	1,4	+ 3,4	0,5	0,7	1,1	1,1	+ 1,3	0,6	0,8	1,2	0,028
BD (mg/dL)	0,5	+ 1,7	0,2	0,3	0,4	0,7	+ 2,4	0,2	0,2	0,4	0,5	+ 0,6	0,2	0,3	0,5	<0,001
BI (mg/dL)	0,7	+ 1,o	0,4	0,5	0,8	0,8	+ 1,2	0,4	0,5	0,8	0,7	+ 0,8	0,4	0,5	0,8	0,227
CRE (g/dL)	1,3	+ 6,4	0,7	0,8	1,o	1,o	+ 0,8	0,7	0,8	1,o	1,6	+ 8,6	0,7	0,8	1,0	0,579
APRI	2,2	+ 6,4	0,4	0,8	2,0	1,8	+ 4,7	0,3	0,6	1,4	2,5	+ 7,43	0,5	1,0	2,3	<0,001
FIB4	3,9	+ 8,4	1,1	1,9	4,3	2,8	+ 3,8	0,9	1,5	2,9	4,7	+ 10,6	1,3	2,3	5,2	<0,001

Table 4 shows the liver profile of all the patients according to whether or not they drank coffee. In the coffee group (*n= 758*) we observed an improvement in the liver profile and in the progression of cirrhosis, as there was a decrease in AST levels (p = 0.004) and total bilirubin (p = 0.034) and platelet and albumin levels increased (p = 0.0054). The TP-INR ratio was not statistically significant.

However, when comparing the APRI and FIB4 calculations, we can see that the group that drinks coffee has better indices than the non-drinkers (p = 0.002 and p = 0.003, respectively).

Table 4 - laboratory aspects according to coffee intake in all patients

	They don't drink coffee						They drink coffee						p
Variable	n=		411 (35%)				n= 758 (65%)						
	average		DP	25%	Median	75%	average		DP	25%	Median	75%	
ALT (IU/L)	75,3	±	133,1	27	44	82	71,0	±	216,3	25	42	71	0,87
AST (IU/L)	77,2	±	166,4	27	44	74	63,0	±	149,1	26	38	64	0,004
FA (IU/L)	103,2	±	60,6	66,	85	119	95,6	±	50,2	65	82,5	107	0,071
GGT (IU/L)	93,9	±	120,3	26	53	111	88,0	±	105,4	27	52	99,5	0,897
PLAQ (mil/mm)^3	163,5	±	87,1	91	161	228	174,0	±	87,9	103,75	174	228,0	0,054
TP-INR	1,1	±	0,3	1	1,1	1,2	1,1	±	0,2	1	1,1	1,2	0,082
ALB (g/dL)	4,1	±	0,6	3,8	4,2	4,6	4,2	±	0,6	4	4,3	4,6	0,013
BT (mg/dL)	1,4	±	3,1	0,6	0,8	1,2	1,2	±	2,1	0,5	0,7	1,2	0,034
BD (mg/dL)	0,6	±	2,0	0,2	0,3	0,5	0,5	±	1,4	0,2	0,3	0,4	0,068
BI (mg/dL)	0,8	±	1,3	0,4	0,5	0,8	0,7	±	0,9	0,4	0,5	0,8	0,093
CRE (g/dL)	1,6	±	9,3	0,7	0,8	1	1,2	±	4,1	0,7	0,8	1	0,435
APRI	2,8	±	9,2	0,5	1	2,3	1,9	±	4,1	0,4	0,7	1,8	0,002
FIB4	4,8	±	12,4	1,2	2,1	5,3	3,4	±	4,9	1,1	1,7	3,9	0,003

Tables 5 and 6 show the liver profile separated by type of hepatitis virus and whether or not coffee was consumed. For B virus carriers who consumed coffee (Table 5), the levels of liver enzymes showed no statistical difference when compared to those who did not consume coffee, i.e. for this group, coffee intake had no hepatoprotective effect.

Table 5 - Laboratory findings according to coffee intake in patients with chronic hepatitis B

Variable	They don't drink coffee n= 171 (33%)					They drink coffee n= 343 (67%)					p
	average	DP	25%	Median	75%	average	DP	25%	Median	75%	
ALT (IU/L)	63,9 ±	157,2	21	32	53	79,8 ±	315,3	19	31	63	0,894
AST (IU/L)	65,9 ±	176,7	23	31	54	67,4 ±	216	22	30	48,5	0,294
FA (IU/L)	96,3 ±	47	66	83	118	96,7 ±	55	63,5	80	104	0,381
GGT (IU/L)	79 ±	119,3	21	36	80,5	75,7 ±	98,1	21	42	79	0,511
PLAQ (mil/mm3)	171,5 ±	82,4	108	177	223	184,1 ±	84,1	126	187	235	0,099
TP-INR	1,2 ±	0,3	1	1,1	1,2	1,1 ±	0,2	1	1,1	1,2	0,411
ALB (g/dL)	4,2 ±	0,7	4	4,3	4,6	4,2 ±	0,6	4	4,4	4,6	0,516
BT (mg/dL)	1,6 ±	4,4	0,6	0,8	1,2	1,3 ±	2,8	0,5	0,7	1,1	0,231
BD (mg/dL)	0,7 ±	2,9	0,1	0,2	0,4	0,6 ±	2,1	0,2	0,2	0,4	0,497
BI (mg/dL)	0,9 ±	1,5	0,4	0,5	0,9	0,7 ±	1	0,3	0,5	0,7	0,155
CRE (g/dL)	0,9 ±	0,5	0,7	0,8	1	1,0 ±	0.9	0,7	0,8	1	0,857
APRI	1,7 ±	3,3	0,3	0,7	1,8	1,8 ±	5,3	0,3	0,6	1,2	0,137
FIB4	3,1 ±	4,2	0,9	1,6	3,7	2,6 ±	3,6	0,9	1,4	2,6	0,179

In Table 6, patients with the C virus showed differences in enzyme levels when compared to the group of patients with the B virus. The ALT and AST enzymes were lower in those who consumed coffee (p = 0.021 and p = 0.005, respectively). APRI and FIB4 calculations were lower and also showed statistical significance for the coffee-drinking group (p = 0.013 for both comparisons).

Albumin levels increased significantly while the other laboratory results also showed a reduction (BD, Creatinine, GGT, FA), but were not statistically significant.

Table 6 - Laboratory findings according to coffee intake in patients with chronic hepatitis C

Variables	Do not drink coffee n= 240 (37%)					They drink coffee n= 415 (63%)					p
	average	DP	25%	Median	75%	average	DP	25%	Median	75%	
ALT (IU/L)	83,6	± 112,7	34,0	60,0	94,5	63,7	± 57,7	32,0	51,0	77,0	0,021
AST (IU/L)	85,2	± 158,6	35,0	52,0	83,3	58,6	± 45,3	30,0	46,0	72,0	0,005
FA (IU/L)	108,1	± 68,4	67,0	85,0	123,0	94,7	± 46,0	67,0	84,0	108,0	0,105
GGT (IU/L)	104,5	± 120,1	34,0	66,0	122,5	98,2	± 110,2	34,0	59,0	127,0	0,653
PLAQ (mil/mm $)^3$	157,7	± 89,9	84,8	147,0	231,5	165,7	± 90,2	90,5	159,0	217,5	0,272
TP-INR	1,1	± 0,2	1,0	1,1	1,2	1,1	± 0,3	1,0	1,1	1,2	0,123
ALB (g/dL)	4,1	± 0,6	3,8	4,2	4,5	4,2	± 0,5	4,0	4,3	4,5	0,006
BT (mg/dL)	1,2	± 1,7	0,6	0,8	1,2	1,1	± 1,1	0,6	0,8	1,2	0,115
BD (mg/dL)	0,5	± 0,9	0,2	0,3	0,5	0,4	± 0,5	0,2	0,3	0,4	0,112
BI (mg/dL)	0,8	± 1,0	0,4	0,6	0,8	0,7	± 0,7	0,4	0,5	0,8	0,413
CRE (g/dL)	2,0	± 12,2	0,7	0,8	1,0	1,3	± 5,6	0,7	0,8	1,0	0,228
APRI	3,6	± 11,6	0,6	1,2	3,2	1,9	± 2,9	0,5	0,9	2,2	0,013
FIB4	6,0	± 15,8	1,4	2,5	6,4	3,9	± 5,7	1,2	2,2	4,6	0,013

Table 7 shows the laboratory data according to daily coffee intake separated according to the amount of coffee ingested (0ml, <100ml and ≥100ml). We can see that there is no statistical difference between the groups when compared according to the amount ingested.

Table 7 - laboratory aspects according to the amount of coffee ingested

Variable	No coffee n=411 (35%)					Drink coffee <100 mL n= 455 (39%)					They drink coffee ≥100mL n= 303 (26%)					P
	average	DP	25%	Median	75%	average	DP	25%	Median	75%	average	DP	25%	Median	75%	
ALT (UI/L)	75,3	+ 133,1	27	44	82	79,5	+ 274,6	25,0	44,0	7530	58,1	+ 60,6	24,0	39,0	69,0	0,341
AST (UI/L)	77,2	+ 166,4	27	44	74	70,8	+ 189,0	26,0	39,0	65,0	50,3	+ 41,3	25,0	36,0	60,0	0,327
FA (UI/L)	103,2	+ 60,6	66,	85	119	94,9	+ 50,8	65,0	82,0	105,0	96,6	+ 49,4	67,0	84,0	107,0	0,297
GGT (UI/L)	93,9	+ 120,3	26	53	111	85,0	+ 101,7	27,0	53,0	98,0	92,6	+ 110,8	26,0	52,0	106,0	0,929
PLAQ (mil/mm)^3	163,5	+ 87,1	91	161	228	171,7	+ 87,7	98,0	170,0	228,0	177,5	+ 88,3	116,0	179,0	225,0	0,427
TP-INR	1,1	+ 0,3	1	1,1	1,2	1,1	+ 0,3	1,0	1,1	1,2	1,1	+ 0,2	1,0	1,1	1,2	0,453
ALB (g/dL)	4,1	+ 0,6	3,8	4,2	4,6	4,2	+ 0,6	4,0	4,3	4,6	4,2	+ 0,5	4,0	4,3	4,6	0,832
BT (mg/dL)	1,4	+ 3,1	0,6	0,8	1,2	1,3	+ 2,2	0,5	0,8	1,2	1,1	+ 1,8	0,5	0,7	1,1	0,227
BD (mg/dL)	0,6	+ 2,0	0,2	0,3	0,5	0,5	+ 1,6	0,2	0,3	0,4	0,4	+ 1,1	0,2	0,2	0,4	0,179
BI (mg/dL)	0,8	+ 1,3	0,4	0,5	0,8	0,7	+ 0,8	0,4	0,5	0,8	0,7	+ 0,9	0,3	0,5	0,7	0,270
CRE (g/dL)	1,6	+ 9,3	0,7	0,8	1	1,3	+ 5,3	0,7	0,8	1,0	1,0	+ 0,8	0,7	0,8	1,0	0,793
APRI	2,8	+ 9,2	0,5	1	2,3	2,1	+ 5,1	0,4	0,8	2,0	1,4	+ 1,9	0,4	0,7	1,6	0,223
FIB4	4,8	+ 12,4	1,2	2,1	5,3	3,7	+ 5,7	1,1	1,8	4,2	2,9	+ 3,3	1,0	1,7	3,2	0,155

4. Discussion

In the last 10 years, many studies have analyzed the effect of coffee on the progression of liver disease. Several meta-analyses , -[105280] have concluded that the greater the amount of coffee ingested, the greater the benefit for the liver. Among the benefits, coffee has an important effect on improving the progression of liver fibrosis, mortality from cirrhosis or the risk of hepatocellular carcinoma. Tables 8, 9 and 10 list some studies on the effects of coffee on hepatitis B, hepatitis C and hepatocellular carcinoma, respectively. The literature shows that coffee can improve the progression of liver disease and improve fibrosis( ).[81]

Our study assessed the benefits that coffee can bring to hepatitis B and C patients by questioning them about their coffee intake. In general, we found that almost 65% of all patients drink coffee and, if we consider gender, women are the ones who consume the most (Table 1). We also saw that the drink may have a hepatoprotective effect by lowering AST levels and improving platelet levels in C virus patients.

Even though percutaneous liver biopsy is considered the "gold standard" for assessing and analyzing the evolution of chronic liver diseases, the use of non-invasive markers to determine the degree of liver fibrosis is a recent alternative that has been widely used in recent years. This group includes the AST-to-platelet ratio index (APRI) and Fibrosis-4 (FIB-4)[77, 82, 83] . In this study, as it was a retrospective study, many patients did not have biopsy data at the time the laboratory tests were taken, so non-invasive methods that were available for diagnosis were used. The APRI and FIB4 calculations also confirm these results, suggesting that in chronic hepatopathies, coffee had a hepatoprotective effect, especially in relation to fibrogenesis markers (Table 4), regardless of the type of virus.

Table 8 - Studies evaluating the impact of coffee on liver outcomes in patients with chronic hepatitis B

Reference	Year	Design	Group	n	Parents	Found
Corrao *et al* (84)	2001	Case-Control	Cases	36	Italy	Coffee can prevent the onset of alcoholic and non-alcoholic cirrhosis
			Control	13		
Goh *et al* (85)	2014	Prospective Cohort		63 275	Singapore	Coffee shows a protective effect on mortality from cirrhosis related to non-viral hepatitis. However, coffee consumption was not related to mortality from HBV cirrhosis.
Inoue *et al* (63)	2009	Prospective Cohort II	HBV	1499	Japan	Drinking coffee can reduce the risk of liver cancer, regardless of whether you have the B or C virus.
Ong *et al* (69)	2011	Transversal		1045	China	Caffeine was not associated with a reduction in fibrosis in B virus-infected patients
Jang *et al* (11)	2013	Case-Control	HCE	408	Korea	The high consumption of coffee was negatively associated with the development of HCC, but in HBV patients, this exposure is reduced in HCC by the dominant role of viral replication
			CLD	626		
			HCC	258		
Leung *et al* (86)	2011	Case-Control	Cases	109	Hong Kong	Moderate coffee consumption in hepatitis B virus carriers reduces the risk of HCC
			Controls	125		

Source: Adapted from Saab *et al*, 2014[81]

Table 9 - Studies evaluating the impact of coffee on liver outcomes in patients with chronic hepatitis C

Reference	Year	Design	Group	n	Parents	Found
Corrao *et al* (84)	2001	Case-Control	Cases	128	Italy	Coffee can prevent the onset of alcoholic and non-alcoholic cirrhosis
			Control	24		
Inoue *et al* (63)	2009	Prospective Cohort II	HCV	1058	Japan	Coffee consumption can reduce the risk of liver cancer, regardless of whether it is B virus or not. C
Freedman *et al* (68)	2009	Retrospective Cohort		766	USA	Coffee reduces the progression of HCV
Freedman *et al* (87)	2011	Retrospective Cohort		885	USA	Coffee is a better predictor of virological response to PegInterferon plus Ribavirin in HCV patients
Modi *et al* (61)	2010	Retrospective Cohort		177	USA	Coffee consumption was associated with a decrease in fibrosis in HCV patients
Costentin *et al* (54)	2011	Transversal		238	France	Caffeine consumption of more than 3 cups a day is associated with a decrease in histological activity.
Carrieri *et al (88)*	2012	Retrospective cohort		601	France	Coffee consumption reduces the risk of insulin resistance in HIV/HCV co-infected patients
Carrieri *et al* (89)	2012	Retrospective cohort		106	France	Coffee consumption alleviates the adverse effects of pegylated Interferon and Ribavirin
Khalaf *et al* (90)	2015	Cross-sectional study	HCV cases (F3/F4-F4)	342	USA	Modest coffee consumption may protect against fibrosis progression in men with HCV
			Controls HCV (F0- F3)	568		
Cardin *et al* (91)	2013	Randomized Study	With coffee	37	Italy	Coffee consumption reduces oxidative stress, increases apoptosis, reduces the risk of disease progression and development into HCC
			No coffee			
Machado *et al* (92)	2014	Cohort	Cases	64	Brazil	Higher caffeine consumption was associated with a reduction in liver fibrosis. The study supports that coffee has a hepatoprotective effect in HCV patients
			Controls	136		
Wakai *et al* (58)	2007	Case-Control	Cases	96	Japan	Coffee is associated with a lower risk of death from HCC in patients with hepatitis C virus
			Controls (HCV+)	420		
			Controls (HCV-)	3024		

Table 10 - Studies evaluating the impact of coffee on chronic liver disease and the risk of hepatocellular carcinoma (HCC)

Reference	Year	Design	Group	n	Parents	Found
La Vecchia et al (93)	1989	Case-Control	Cases	151	Italy	No association between coffee and liver cancer
			Controls	1944		
Ohfuji et al (94)	2006	Case-Control	Cases (HCV)	73	Japan	Inverse association between coffee intake and liver cancer incidence
			Controls	253		
Ohishi et al (95)	2008	Case-Control	Cases	224	Japan	Daily consumption was associated with a decreased risk of HCC
			Controls	644		
Gelatti et al (66)	2005	Case-Control	Cases	250	Italy	Inverse association between coffee and the incidence of HCC
			Controls	500		
Gallus et al (65)	2002	Case-Control	Cases	501	Italy	Inverse association between coffee and the incidence of HCC
			Controls	1552		
Johnson et al (12)	2011	Retrospective Cohort		61 321	China	Coffee can reduce the risk of HCC
Kuper et al (96)	2000	Case-Control	Cases	333	Greece	Coffee was not positively associated with the incidence of HCC
			Controls	360		
Shimazu et al (97)	2005	Prospective Cohort I		22 204	Japan	Inverse (dose-dependent) association between coffee and the incidence of HCC
		Prospective Cohort II		38 703		
Montella et al (98)	2007	Case-Control	Cases	185	Italy	Inverse association between caffeinated coffee and HCC
			Controls	412		
Tanaka et al (64)	2007	Case-Control	Cases	209	Japan	Inverse association (dose-dependent) between coffee use particularly among community and CLD controls
			Controls	1308		
			Community	275		
			Hospital	381		
			CLD			
Hu et al (99)	2008	Prospective Cohort		60 323	Finland	Inverse dose-dependent association between coffee and the risk of HCC
Inoue et al (63)	2009	Prospective Cohort		18 815	Japan	Coffee consumption can reduce the risk of liver cancer, regardless of the type of hepatitis virus

Study	Year	Study design	Sample		Location	Conclusion
						(HBV or HCV).
Aleksandrova *et al* 2015 (100)		Case-Control	Cases Controls	125 250	Cities of Europe	Inverse association between coffee intake and risk of HCC
Lai *et al* (101)	2013	Prospective Cohort		27 037	Finland	Coffee intake was inversely associated with the incidence of liver cancer and mortality from chronic liver disease.
Bamia *et al* (102)	2015	Case-Control	Cases Controls	125 250	European countries	Inverse association between coffee intake and risk of HCC
Petrick *et al* (103)	2015	Cohort	HCC ICC	860 260	USA	Consuming a large amount of coffee was associated with a lower risk of HCC

Source: Adapted from Saab *et al*, 2014[81]

For chronic hepatitis C, Lin *et al* [83] carried out a large meta-analysis which suggests that the APRI index for staging fibrosis has a moderate degree of accuracy. Xiao *et al* (104) also in a review and meta-analysis concluded that APRI and FIB-4 for hepatitis B can identify fibrosis with a moderate degree of sensitivity and accuracy. However, in another meta-analysis for chronic hepatitis B, Jin *et al* [77] suggest that the APRI index for staging fibrosis has limitations in this group of patients. In our study, APRI and FIB4 calculations showed a reduction in the general group of patients with hepatitis C, suggesting that coffee also has a beneficial effect in this group of patients, but further studies involving cirrhotic patients would be necessary to clarify these results.

In our study, the medians of the liver enzymes ALT ($p < 0.001$), AST ($p < 0.001$) and GGT ($p < 0.001$) and the medians of APRI ($p < 0.001$) and FIB4 ($p < 0.001$) have lower values for patients with chronic hepatitis caused by HBV when compared to the C virus, suggesting groups with different stages of the disease, with the group of patients with hepatitis C having a more advanced stage of the disease. When assessing alcohol consumption among the patients, we found that male patients consumed more alcohol ($p<0.001$) than female patients (Table 1), and the frequency of alcohol consumption was higher among patients with chronic hepatitis B ($p<0.001$) (Table 2).

When evaluating other habits, such as smoking, for example, 18% of all patients are smokers. Tobacco may reduce the effect of coffee on liver disease[55] possibly by inducing the CYP enzyme to excrete bioactive compounds, but more studies are needed to understand this relationship.

With regard to platelets, we saw that coffee drinkers had higher levels. Albumin also showed an increase in coffee drinkers, but only the C virus group showed statistically significant data. For the Hepatitis B virus carrier group, there was no statistical significance for liver enzymes, only for damage markers, which were lower in coffee drinkers. In the group with Hepatitis C, both the enzymes and the markers of damage were reduced when drinking coffee, and alcohol intake was also lower.

The number of studies involving hepatitis B virus carriers is still scarce, showing only the protective effect of coffee on the risk of developing hepatocellular carcinoma, but no evidence of lower mortality from cirrhosis related to HBV[85] (Table 8). Thus, although the role of coffee is well defined for the group of patients with hepatitis C (Table 9) and on the risk of developing hepatocellular carcinoma (Table 10), its role on fibrogenesis in hepatitis B is still unclear, with publications showing conflicting results (Table 8). Our study confirmed that for patients with chronic hepatitis B, coffee consumption had no beneficial effect on transaminases or fibrogenesis as assessed by APRI or FIB4 (Table 5).

Overall, it was observed that for coffee drinkers, the beverage had a hepatoprotective effect by decreasing the levels of liver enzymes. The APRI and FIB4 calculations also confirmed these results, even for consumption with both types of virus. We can therefore conclude that coffee had a hepatoprotective effect and improved the progression of the disease in these groups of patients with liver disease. There was no statistical significance in the TP-INR analysis.

We can observe a slight increase in platelet values, which could indicate an improvement in the inflammatory condition of liver disease, but a more in-depth analysis of the volume ingested should be carried out to elucidate the ideal volume of coffee to enhance its beneficial effect.

In hepatitis B, liver enzymes have lower values for both coffee drinkers and non-coffee drinkers compared to the C virus, but the data was statistically significant for enzymes in the group of patients with the C virus. Goh *et al* (85) described that alcohol consumption has a strong positive association between the amount of alcohol consumed and the risk of mortality from cirrhosis. For the Hepatitis B virus carrier group, there was no statistical significance for liver enzymes, only for markers of damage, which were lower in coffee drinkers. In our study, it is possible that alcohol intake could hinder the action of the polyphenols present in coffee, since alcohol consumption in the group of patients with hepatitis B was higher than in the hepatitis C group. In the group with hepatitis C, it was observed that both enzymes and fibrosis markers (APRI and FIB-4) were reduced when coffee was consumed and alcohol intake was also lower in this group.

This study has some limitations. Firstly, only laboratory tests were evaluated. Especially for hepatitis B, it would be interesting to include other tests to assess fibrosis, such as liver biopsy, imaging tests or hepatic elastometry. Secondly, no analysis was carried out considering the effect of alcohol and antiviral treatment, which are known to worsen and improve the progression of liver disease respectively. Thirdly, there were no analyses evaluating smoking either. The positive points are that this is the first study with a significant number of patients with chronic hepatitis B and C to evaluate coffee consumption and its effect on liver enzymes and the APRI and FIB4 indices. For chronic hepatitis C, this is the first study to evaluate the APRI and FIB4 indices and coffee consumption.

5. Conclusion

Among patients with chronic liver disease caused by HBV and HCV, 758/1,169 (65%) are coffee drinkers.

Patients with chronic hepatitis C who drink coffee have lower ALT (p=0.021), AST (p=0.005), APRI (p=0.013) and FIB4 (p=0.013) levels and higher albumin levels (p=0.006). The same was not observed for patients with chronic hepatitis B.

Coffee intake is associated with a reduction in liver enzymes and seems to be directly linked to a decrease in APRI and FIB4 values in patients with chronic hepatitis C. The same is not observed for chronic hepatitis B.

5. Bibliographical references

1. Antia FP, Abraham P. Clinical Dietetics and Nutrition. 4ª ed. England: Oxford University Press; 1997. 524 p.

2. Fox GP, Wu A, Yiran L, Force L. Variation in caffeine concentration in single coffee beans. J Agric Food Chem. 2013;61(45):10772-8.

3. Simoes J, Nunes FM, Domingues MR, Coimbra MA. Extractability and structure of spent coffee ground polysaccharides by roasting pre-treatments. Carbohydr Polym. 2013;97(1):81-9.

4. Valko M, Leibfritz D, Moncol J, Cronin MT, Mazur M, Telser J. Free radicals and antioxidants in normal physiological functions and human disease. Int J Biochem Cell Biol. 2007;39(1):44-84.

5. Doo T, Morimoto Y, Steinbrecher A, Kolonel LN, Maskarinec G. Coffee intake and risk of type 2 diabetes: the Multiethnic Cohort. Public Health Nutr. 2013:1-9.

6. Cadden IS, Partovi N, Yoshida EM. Review article: possible beneficial effects of coffee on liver disease and function. Aliment Pharmacol Ther. 2007;26(1):1-8.

7. Danielsson J, Kangastupa P, Laatikainen T, Aalto M, Niemela O. Dose- and gender-dependent interactions between coffee consumption and serum GGT activity in alcohol consumers. Alcohol Alcohol. 2013;48(3):303-7.

8. Cano-Marquina A, Tarin JJ, Cano A. The impact of coffee on health. Maturitas. 2013;75(1):7-21.

9. Butt MS, Sultan MT. Coffee and its consumption: benefits and risks. Crit Rev Food Sci Nutr. 2011;51(4):363-73.

10. Sang LX, Chang B, Li XH, Jiang M. Consumption of coffee associated with reduced risk of liver cancer: a meta-analysis. BMC Gastroenterol. 2013;13:34.

11. Jang ES, Jeong SH, Lee SH, Hwang SH, Ahn SY, Lee J, et al. The effect of coffee consumption on the development of hepatocellular carcinoma in hepatitis B virus endemic area. Liver Int. 2013;33(7):1092-9.

12. Johnson S, Koh WP, Wang R, Govindarajan S, Yu MC, Yuan JM. Coffee consumption

and reduced risk of hepatocellular carcinoma: findings from the Singapore Chinese Health Study. Cancer Causes Control. 2011;22(3):503-10.

13. Cagliani LR, Pellegrino G, Giugno G, Consonni R. Quantification of Coffea arabica and Coffea canephora var. robusta in roasted and ground coffee blends. Talanta. 2013;106:169-73.

14. Vilela DM. In vitro selection of starter cultures for fermentation of coffee fruits (coffea arabicaL.) processed by dry and semi-dry methods. Lavras: Federal University of Lavras; 2011.

15. Toci A, Farah A, Trugo LC. Effect of the decaffeination process with dichloromethane on the chemical composition of Arabica and Robusta coffees before and after roasting2006; 29:[965-71 pp.].

16. Monteiro MC, Trugo LC. Determination of bioactive compounds in commercial samples of roasted coffee2005; 28:[637-41 pp.].

17. Higdon JV, Frei B. Coffee and health: a review of recent human research. Crit Rev Food Sci Nutr. 2006;46(2):101-23.

18. Kaiser N, Birkholz D, Colomban S, Navarini L, Engelhardt UH. A new method for the preparative isolation of chlorogenic acid lactones from coffee and model roasts of 5-caffeoylquinic acid. J Agric Food Chem. 2013;61(28):6937-41.

19. Lang R, Yagar EF, Wahl A, Beusch A, Dunkel A, Dieminger N, et al. Quantitative studies on roast kinetics for bioactives in coffee. J Agric Food Chem. 2013;61(49):12123-8.

20. Park JB. Isolation and quantification of major chlorogenic acids in three major instant coffee brands and their potential effects on H2O2-induced mitochondrial membrane depolarization and apoptosis in PC-12 cells. Food Funct. 2013;4(11):1632-8.

21. D'Amelio N, De Angelis E, Navarini L, Schievano E, Mammi S. Green coffee oil analysis by high-resolution nuclear magnetic resonance spectroscopy. Talanta. 2013;110:118-27.

22. Cavin C, Holzhaeuser D, Scharf G, Constable A, Huber WW, Schilter B. Cafestol and kahweol, two coffee specific diterpenes with anticarcinogenic activity. Food Chem Toxicol. 2002;40(8):1155-63.

23. Lee KJ, Choi JH, Jeong HG. Hepatoprotective and antioxidant effects of the coffee

diterpenes kahweol and cafestol on carbon tetrachloride-induced liver damage in mice. Food Chem Toxicol. 2007;45(11):2118-25.

24. Cavin C, Mace K, Offord EA, Schilter B. Protective effects of coffee diterpenes against aflatoxin B1-induced genotoxicity: mechanisms in rat and human cells. Food Chem Toxicol. 2001;39(6):549-56.

25. Corrêa TA, Rogero MM, Mioto BM, Tarasoutchi D, Tuda VL, César LA, et al. Paper-filtered coffee increases cholesterol and inflammation biomarkers independent of roasting degree: a clinical trial. Nutrition. 2013;29(7-8):977-81.

26. RODARTE MP, ABRAHAO SA, PEREIRA RGFA, MALTA MR. NON-VOLATILE COMPOUNDS IN COFFEES FROM THE SOUTHERN REGION OF MINAS GERAIS SUBJECTED TO DIFFERENT ROASTING POINTS2009; VOL.33:[1366-71 PP.].

27. Crozier TW, Stalmach A, Lean ME, Crozier A. Espresso coffees, caffeine and chlorogenic acid intake: potential health implications. Food Funct. 2012;3(1):30-3.

28. Organization I-IC. About Coffee England [

29. Abrahao SA, Pereira RGFA, Lima AR, Ferreira EB, Malta MR. **Bioactive compounds in whole bean and decaffeinated coffee and beverage sensory quality**. In: Pereira RGFA, Lima AR, Ferreira EB, Malta MR, editors. Brasilia: Pesquisa Agropecuària Brasileira; 2008. p. 1799=804.

30. Krakowian D, Skiba D, Kudelski A, Pilawa B, Ramos P, Adamczyk J, et al. Application of EPR spectroscopy to the examination of pro-oxidant activity of coffee. Food Chem. 2014;151:110-9.

31. Lang R, Fromme T, Beusch A, Wahl A, Klingenspor M, Hofmann T. 2-O-β-D-Glucopyranosyl-carboxyatractyligenin from Coffea L. inhibits adenine nucleotide translocase in isolated mitochondria but is quantitatively degraded during coffee roasting. Phytochemistry. 2013;93:124-35.

32. Yen WJ, Wang BS, Chang LW, Duh PD. Antioxidant properties of roasted coffee residues. J Agric Food Chem. 2005;53(7):2658-63.

33. Lang R, Dieminger N, Beusch A, Lee YM, Dunkel A, Suess B, et al. Bioappearance and pharmacokinetics of bioactives upon coffee consumption. Anal Bioanal Chem.

2013;405(26):8487-503.

34. Masi C, Dinnella C, Barnabà M, Navarini L, Monteleone E. Sensory properties of under-roasted coffee beverages. J Food Sci. 2013;78(8):S1290-300.

35. Bicho NC, Leitao AE, Ramalho JC, de Alvarenga NB, Lidon FC. Impact of roasting time on the sensory profile of arabica and robusta coffee. Ecol Food Nutr. 2013;52(2):163-77.

36. SINDICAFÉ - Union of Coffee Industries of the State of Sao Paulo. Preparation Tips [2016]

37. ABIC - Brazilian Coffee Industries Association. Consumer Rio de Janeiro [2016]

38. Valko M, Rhodes CJ, Moncol J, Izakovic M, Mazur M. Free radicals, metals and antioxidants in oxidative stress-induced cancer. Chem Biol Interact. 2006;160(1):1- 40.

39. B0hn SK, Blomhoff R, Paur I. Coffee and cancer risk, epidemiological evidence, and molecular mechanisms. Mol Nutr Food Res. 2014;58(5):915-30.

40. Borges F, Fernandes E, Roleira F. Progress towards the discovery of xanthine oxidase inhibitors. Curr Med Chem. 2002;9(2):195-217.

41. Coleman MD. Human Drug Metabolism: An Introduction. England2005.

42. Orellana M, Guajardo V. [Cytochrome P450 activity and its alteration in different diseases]. Rev Med Chil. 2004;132(1):85-94.

43. Faber MS, Jetter A, Fuhr U. Assessment of CYP1A2 activity in clinical practice: why, how, and when? Basic Clin Pharmacol Toxicol. 2005;97(3):125-34.

44. Gressner OA. Less Smad2 is good for you! A scientific update on coffee's liver benefits. Hepatology. 2009;50(3):970-8.

45. Klemmer I, Yagi S, Gressner OA. Oral application of 1,7-dimethylxanthine (paraxanthine) attenuates the formation of experimental cholestatic liver fibrosis. Hepatol Res. 2011;41(11):1094-109.

46. Eteng MU, Eyong EU, Akpanyung EO, Agiang MA, Aremu CY. Recent advances in caffeine and theobromine toxicities: a review. Plant Foods Hum Nutr. 1997;51(3):231-43.

47. EUFIC - The European Food Information Council. Caffeine and Energy Drinks [2016]

48. Scalbert A, Johnson IT, Saltmarsh M. Polyphenols: antioxidants and beyond. Am J Clin Nutr. 2005;81(1 Suppl):215S-7S.

49. Killer SC, Blannin AK, Jeukendrup AE. No evidence of dehydration with moderate daily coffee intake: a counterbalanced cross-over study in a free-living population. PLoS One. 2014;9(1):e84154.

50. Daglia M, Tarsi R, Papetti A, Grisoli P, Dacarro C, Pruzzo C, et al. Antiadhesive effect of green and roasted coffee on Streptococcus mutans' adhesive properties on saliva-coated hydroxyapatite beads. J Agric Food Chem. 2002;50(5):1225-9.

51. Malerba S, Turati F, Galeone C, Pelucchi C, Verga F, La Vecchia C, et al. A meta-analysis of prospective studies of coffee consumption and mortality for all causes, cancers and cardiovascular diseases. Eur J Epidemiol. 2013;28(7):527-39.

52. Ding M, Bhupathiraju SN, Satija A, van Dam RM, Hu FB. Long-term coffee consumption and risk of cardiovascular disease: a systematic review and a doseresponse meta-analysis of prospective cohort studies. Circulation. 2014;129(6):643- 59.

53. Uiterwaal CS, Verschuren WM, Bueno-de-Mesquita HB, Ocké M, Geleijnse JM, Boshuizen HC, et al. Coffee intake and incidence of hypertension. Am J Clin Nutr. 2007;85(3):718-23.

54. Costentin CE, Roudot-Thoraval F, Zafrani ES, Medkour F, Pawlotsky JM, Mallat A, et al. Association of caffeine intake and histological features of chronic hepatitis C. J Hepatol. 2011;54(6):1123-9.

55. Aubin HJ, Laureaux C, Zerah F, Tilikete S, Vernier F, Vallat B, et al. Joint influence of alcohol, tobacco, and coffee on biological markers of heavy drinking in alcoholics. Biol Psychiatry. 1998;44(7):638-43.

56. Wadhawan M, Anand AC. Coffee and Liver Disease. J Clin Exp Hepatol. 2016;6(1):40-6.

57. Inoue M, Yoshimi I, Sobue T, Tsugane S, Group JS. Influence of coffee drinking on subsequent risk of hepatocellular carcinoma: a prospective study in Japan. J Natl Cancer Inst. 2005;97(4):293-300.

58. Wakai K, Kurozawa Y, Shibata A, Fujita Y, Kotani K, Ogimoto I, et al. Liver cancer risk,

coffee, and hepatitis C virus infection: a nested case-control study in Japan. Br J Cancer. 2007;97(3):426-8.

59. Shim SG, Jun DW, Kim EK, Saeed WK, Lee KN, Lee HL, et al. Caffeine attenuates liver fibrosis via defective adhesion of hepatic stellate cells in cirrhotic model. J Gastroenterol Hepatol. 2013;28(12):1877-84.

60. Arauz J, Moreno MG, Cortés-Reynosa P, Salazar EP, Muriel P. Coffee attenuates fibrosis by decreasing the expression of TGF-β and CTGF in a murine model of liver damage. J Appl Toxicol. 2013;33(9):970-9.

61. Modi AA, Feld JJ, Park Y, Kleiner DE, Everhart JE, Liang TJ, et al. Increased caffeine consumption is associated with reduced hepatic fibrosis. Hepatology. 2010;51(1):201-9.

62. Jodynis-Liebert J, Flieger J, Matuszewska A, Juszczyk J. Serum metabolite/caffeine ratios as a test for liver function. J Clin Pharmacol. 2004;44(4):338-47.

63. Inoue M, Kurahashi N, Iwasaki M, Shimazu T, Tanaka Y, Mizokami M, et al. Effect of coffee and green tea consumption on the risk of liver cancer: cohort analysis by hepatitis virus infection status. Cancer Epidemiol Biomarkers Prev. 2009;18(6):1746-53.

64. Tanaka K, Hara M, Sakamoto T, Higaki Y, Mizuta T, Eguchi Y, et al. Inverse association between coffee drinking and the risk of hepatocellular carcinoma: a case-control study in Japan. Cancer Sci. 2007;98(2):214-8.

65. Gallus S, Bertuzzi M, Tavani A, Bosetti C, Negri E, La Vecchia C, et al. Does coffee protect against hepatocellular carcinoma? Br J Cancer. 2002;87(9):956-9.

66. Gelatti U, Covolo L, Franceschini M, Pirali F, Tagger A, Ribero ML, et al. Coffee consumption reduces the risk of hepatocellular carcinoma independently of its aetiology: a case-control study. J Hepatol. 2005;42(4):528-34.

67. Tanida I, Shirasago Y, Suzuki R, Abe R, Wakita T, Hanada K, et al. Inhibitory Effects of Caffeic Acid, a Coffee-Related Organic Acid, on the Propagation of Hepatitis C Virus. Jpn J Infect Dis. 2015;68(4):268-75.

68. Freedman ND, Everhart JE, Lindsay KL, Ghany MG, Curto TM, Shiffman ML, et al. Coffee intake is associated with lower rates of liver disease progression in chronic hepatitis C. Hepatology. 2009;50(5):1360-9.

69. Ong A, Wong VW, Wong GL, Chan HL. The effect of caffeine and alcohol consumption on liver fibrosis - a study of 1045 Asian hepatitis B patients using transient elastography. Liver Int. 2011;31(7):1047-53.

70. Wang GF, Shi LP, Ren YD, Liu QF, Liu HF, Zhang RJ, et al. Anti-hepatitis B virus activity of chlorogenic acid, quinic acid and caffeic acid in vivo and in vitro. Antiviral Res. 2009;83(2):186-90.

71. Abrahao SA, Pereira RG, de Sousa RV, Lima AR, Crema GP, Barros BS. Influence of coffee brew in metabolic syndrome and type 2 diabetes. Plant Foods Hum Nutr. 2013;68(2):184-9.

72. Gavrieli A, Fragopoulou E, Mantzoros CS, Yannakoulia M. Gender and body mass index modify the effect of increasing amounts of caffeinated coffee on postprandial glucose and insulin concentrations; a randomized, controlled, clinical trial. Metabolism. 2013;62(8):1099-106.

73. Bambha K, Wilson LA, Unalp A, Loomba R, Neuschwander-Tetri BA, Brunt EM, et al. Coffee consumption in NAFLD patients with lower insulin resistance is associated with lower risk of severe fibrosis. Liver Int. 2013.

74. Jiang X, Zhang D, Jiang W. Coffee and caffeine intake and incidence of type 2 diabetes mellitus: a meta-analysis of prospective studies. Eur J Nutr. 2014;53(1):25- 38.

75. Bravi F, Bosetti C, Tavani A, Gallus S, La Vecchia C. Coffee reduces risk for hepatocellular carcinoma: an updated meta-analysis. Clin Gastroenterol Hepatol. 2013;11(11):1413-21.e1.

76. Sterling RK, Lissen E, Clumeck N, Sola R, Correa MC, Montaner J, et al. Development of a simple noninvasive index to predict significant fibrosis in patients with HIV/HCV coinfection. Hepatology. 2006;43(6):1317-25.

77. Jin W, Lin Z, Xin Y, Jiang X, Dong Q, Xuan S. Diagnostic accuracy of the aspartate aminotransferase-to-platelet ratio index for the prediction of hepatitis B- related fibrosis: a leading meta-analysis. BMC Gastroenterol. 2012;12:14.

78. Yosry A, Fouad R, Alem SA, Elsharkawy A, El-Sayed M, Asem N, et al. FibroScan, APRI, FIB4, and GUCI: Role in prediction of fibrosis and response to therapy in Egyptian patients with HCV infection. Arab J Gastroenterol. 2016;17(2):78- 83.

79. Zeng DW, Dong J, Liu YR, Jiang JJ, Zhu YY. Noninvasive models for assessment of liver fibrosis in patients with chronic hepatitis B virus infection. World J Gastroenterol. 2016;22(29):6663-72.

80. Jiang W, Wu Y, Jiang X. Coffee and caffeine intake and breast cancer risk: an updated dose-response meta-analysis of 37 published studies. Gynecol Oncol. 2013;129(3):620-9.

81. Saab S, Mallam D, Cox GA, Tong MJ. Impact of coffee on liver diseases: a systematic review. Liver Int. 2014;34(4):495-504.

82. Wai CT, Greenson JK, Fontana RJ, Kalbfleisch JD, Marrero JA, Conjeevaram HS, et al. A simple noninvasive index can predict both significant fibrosis and cirrhosis in patients with chronic hepatitis C. Hepatology. 2003;38(2):518-26.

83. Lin ZH, Xin YN, Dong QJ, Wang Q, Jiang XJ, Zhan SH, et al. Performance of the aspartate aminotransferase-to-platelet ratio index for the staging of hepatitis C- related fibrosis: an updated meta-analysis. Hepatology. 2011;53(3):726-36.

84. Corrao G, Zambon A, Bagnardi V, D'Amicis A, Klatsky A, Group CS. Coffee, caffeine, and the risk of liver cirrhosis. Ann Epidemiol. 2001;11(7):458-65.

85. Goh GB, Chow WC, Wang R, Yuan JM, Koh WP. Coffee, alcohol and other beverages in relation to cirrhosis mortality: the Singapore Chinese Health Study. Hepatology. 2014;60(2):661-9.

86. Leung WW, Ho SC, Chan HL, Wong V, Yeo W, Mok TS. Moderate coffee consumption reduces the risk of hepatocellular carcinoma in hepatitis B chronic carriers: a case-control study. J Epidemiol Community Health. 2011;65(6):556-8.

87. Freedman ND, Curto TM, Lindsay KL, Wright EC, Sinha R, Everhart JE, et al. Coffee consumption is associated with response to peginterferon and ribavirin therapy in patients with chronic hepatitis C. Gastroenterology. 2011;140(7):1961-9.

88. Carrieri MP, Sogni P, Cohen J, Loko MA, Winnock M, Spire B. Elevated coffee consumption and reduced risk of insulin resistance in HIV-HCV coinfected patients (HEPAVIH ANRS CO-13). Hepatology. 2012;56(5):2010.

89. Carrieri MP, Cohen J, Salmon-Ceron D, Winnock M. Coffee consumption and reduced self-reported side effects in HIV-HCV co-infected patients during PEG-IFN and ribavirin

treatment: results from ANRS CO13 HEPAVIH. J Hepatol. 2012;56(3):745-7.

90. Khalaf N, White D, Kanwal F, Ramsey D, Mittal S, Tavakoli-Tabasi S, et al. Coffee and Caffeine Are Associated With Decreased Risk of Advanced Hepatic Fibrosis Among Patients With Hepatitis C. Clin Gastroenterol Hepatol. 2015;13(8):1521-31.e3.

91. Cardin R, Piciocchi M, Martines D, Scribano L, Petracco M, Farinati F. Effects of coffee consumption in chronic hepatitis C: a randomized controlled trial. Dig Liver Dis. 2013;45(6):499-504.

92. Machado SR, Parise ER, de Carvalho L. Coffee has hepatoprotective benefits in Brazilian patients with chronic hepatitis C even in lower daily consumption than in American and European populations. Braz J Infect Dis. 2014;18(2):170-6.

93. La Vecchia C, Ferraroni M, Negri E, D'Avanzo B, Decarli A, Levi F, et al. Coffee consumption and digestive tract cancers. Cancer Res. 1989;49(4):1049-51.

94. Ohfuji S, Fukushima W, Tanaka T, Habu D, Tamori A, Sakaguchi H, et al. Coffee consumption and reduced risk of hepatocellular carcinoma among patients with chronic type C liver disease: A case-control study. Hepatol Res. 2006;36(3):201-8.

95. Ohishi W, Fujiwara S, Cologne JB, Suzuki G, Akahoshi M, Nishi N, et al. Risk factors for hepatocellular carcinoma in a Japanese population: a nested case-control study. Cancer Epidemiol Biomarkers Prev. 2008;17(4):846-54.

96. Kuper H, Tzonou A, Kaklamani E, Hsieh CC, Lagiou P, Adami HO, et al. Tobacco smoking, alcohol consumption and their interaction in the causation of hepatocellular carcinoma. Int J Cancer. 2000;85(4):498-502.

97. Shimazu T, Tsubono Y, Kuriyama S, Ohmori K, Koizumi Y, Nishino Y, et al. Coffee consumption and the risk of primary liver cancer: pooled analysis of two prospective studies in Japan. Int J Cancer. 2005;116(1):150-4.

98. Montella M, Polesel J, La Vecchia C, Dal Maso L, Crispo A, Crovatto M, et al. Coffee and tea consumption and risk of hepatocellular carcinoma in Italy. Int J Cancer. 2007;120(7):1555-9.

99. Hu G, Tuomilehto J, Pukkala E, Hakulinen T, Antikainen R, Vartiainen E, et al. Joint effects of coffee consumption and serum gamma-glutamyltransferase on the risk of liver

cancer. Hepatology. 2008;48(1):129-36.

100. Aleksandrova K, Bamia C, Drogan D, Lagiou P, Trichopoulou A, Jenab M, et al. The association of coffee intake with liver cancer risk is mediated by biomarkers of inflammation and hepatocellular injury: data from the European Prospective Investigation into Cancer and Nutrition. Am J Clin Nutr. 2015;102(6):1498-508.

101. Lai GY, Weinstein SJ, Albanes D, Taylor PR, McGlynn KA, Virtamo J, et al. The association of coffee intake with liver cancer incidence and chronic liver disease mortality in male smokers. Br J Cancer. 2013;109(5):1344-51.

102. Bamia C, Lagiou P, Jenab M, Trichopoulou A, Fedirko V, Aleksandrova K, et al. Coffee, tea and decaffeinated coffee in relation to hepatocellular carcinoma in a European population: multicenter, prospective cohort study. Int J Cancer. 2015;136(8):1899-908.

103. Petrick JL, Freedman ND, Graubard BI, Sahasrabuddhe VV, Lai GY, Alavanja MC, et al. Coffee Consumption and Risk of Hepatocellular Carcinoma and Intrahepatic Cholangiocarcinoma by Sex: The Liver Cancer Pooling Project. Cancer Epidemiol Biomarkers Prev. 2015;24(9):1398-406.

104. Xiao G, Yang J, Yan L. Comparison of diagnostic accuracy of aspartate aminotransferase to platelet ratio index and fibrosis-4 index for detecting liver fibrosis in adult patients with chronic hepatitis B virus infection: a systemic review and metaanalysis. Hepatology. 2015;61(1):292-302.

More
Books!

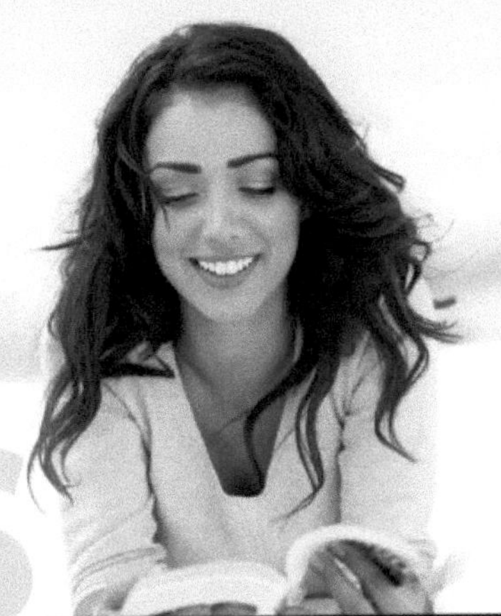

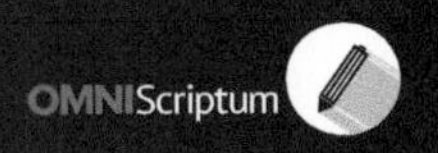

info@omniscriptum.com
www.omniscriptum.com
OMNIScriptum

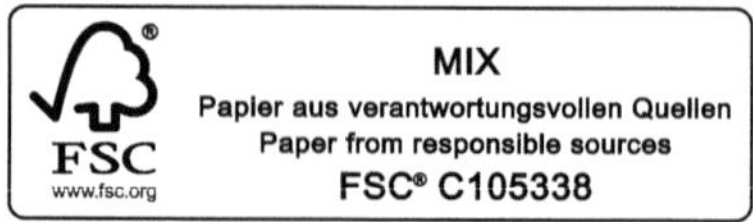

Printed by Books on Demand GmbH, Norderstedt / Germany